How to Get Rid of Cellulite Fast

310 Effective Anti Cellulite Treatment Tips

ADAM COLTON

Published by BizMove
www.bizmove.com

Disclaimer

All the content found in this book was created for informational purposes only. The Content is not intended to be a substitute for professional medical advice, diagnosis, or treatment. Always seek the advice of your physician or other qualified health provider with any questions you may have regarding a medical condition. Never disregard professional medical advice or delay in seeking it because of something you have read in this book.

ISBN: 1979371253
ISBN- 978-1979371254

310 Effective Anti Cellulite Treatment Tips

Cellulite is fat that collects in pockets just below the surface of the skin. It forms around the hips, thighs, and buttocks. Cellulite deposits cause the skin to look dimpled.

Cellulite may be more visible than fat deeper in the body. Everyone has layers of fat under the skin, so even thin people can have cellulite. Collagen fibers that connect fat to the skin may stretch, break down, or pull tight. This allows fat cells to bulge out.

Your genes may play a part in whether or not you have cellulite. Other factors may include:

- Your diet
- How your body burns energy
- Hormone changes
- Dehydration

Despite what the media or popular opinion may have you believing, cellulite is a common problem, even for celebrities. Even if you eat well or exercise regularly, you may notice dimpled skin on your legs or buttocks. Read on for tips on getting rid of that pesky cellulite to regain confidence.

1. Try using your hands to knead the areas of your body affected by cellulite problems. This may sound weird, but in fact that kneading helps circulate blood through your body. This, in turn, helps your body break down all of those ugly fat deposits that you are worrying over.

2. To reduce the appearance of cellulite, make sure you exercise on a regular basis. Make sure you work up a good sweat when you exercise. Sweating helps expel toxins from the body through the skin. Exercise also improves your body's appearance by toning and tightening, so you look better even if you have cellulite.

3. To help minimize the appearance of cellulite on the skin, consider taking action to improve the circulation in the affected areas. By massaging the skin vigorously with a hand or with an electric massage tool, it is possible to accomplish this goal with ease. The bumpy look of the cellulite will soon be far less noticeable.

4. Minimize the appearance of cellulite by limiting the amount of skin thinning cream you use. Using skin thinning creams, like steroid, on areas of cellulite will make the cellulite more obvious. This is due to your skin being thinner and making the dimples under your skin more

noticeable. Also, any imperfections in the skin will be more visible.

5. Want to get rid of that pesky cellulite? Rub some coffee grounds into the area. Give it a good, deep massage and allow the coffee to exfoliate the top layers of skin. Add a little olive oil for lubrication and to ensure the coffee doesn't just fall off all over your floor.

6. Smoking can contribute to cellulite. It is a known fact that smoking speeds up the aging process. The faster you age, the more likely you are to begin seeing cellulite form. If you quit, your skin will become thicker, your body will become healthier and you will be able to battle your cellulite more effectively.

7. Water will help you decrease the chances of problems with cellulite. The more water you drink, the healthier your skin is and the less likely you will be to suffer from cellulite. Water consumption plays a big role in a healthy diet, so drink up your water and you will be healthier overall.

8. Water is essential in keeping your body looking lean, but do not drink too much. Excess water can make you feel bloated, and it can result in

swelling under the cellulite. Drink no more than one and one-half liters for the optimal hydration of your body without over doing it.

9. Beat cellulite through massages. There are many benefits from getting a massage, including promoting circulation, lymphatic drainage, and reducing stress. All of these factors play a role in cellulite, so by getting a massage, you are helping reduce cellulite. Just make sure you are getting massages from a professional who knows what they are doing.

10. Invest in some good anti-cellulite cream. There are plenty of creams out there promising miracles. While there's no magic cream that can erase your cellulite, there are products that can help. A good anti-cellulite cream can firm your skin while providing it with nutrients it needs. Compare product reviews to find something that works for you.

11. So, you want to get rid of your cellulite and you are thinking about sinking a ton of money having your problem areas liposuctioned. Yes, liposuction is a surgical procedure which removes fat. However, it removes deep fat, not the cellulite fat which is just below the skin's surface. In some cases, liposuction actually

creates more dimpling of the skin and worsen the appearance of your cellulite.

12. Want to quickly get all eyes away from your cellulite? Brush a shiny bronzer up and down the front of your legs where they are tight and cellulite-free. This will draw the eye to the front of your body and away from your problem areas, ensuring only the best of you is shown off.

13. To address your cellulite problem, eat foods that are make your skin cells stronger. Extra cellulite makes your skin look bumpy and uneven. Foods high in lecithin strengthen your skin cells and are effective in getting rid of extra cellulite. Include in your diet plenty of apples, spinach, cauliflower, eggs, and soy.

14. Looking to slim down your body and get rid of cellulite? Consider playing a sport. The harder you work, the more fat you burn, and that is exactly what cellulite is made of. If you don't have any fat, you won't have cellulite either, so go join a team and have fun!

15. Try doing some yoga. Yoga is noted for reducing stress, which will help your metabolism. It will also regulate your hormones to a more harmonious state. Yoga also helps to increase

blood flow and tones muscles. All of the benefits work together to fight cellulite and keep it from returning.

16. To return your dermal cells to their original strength, eat foods that are high in lecithin. This means enjoying more apples, fresh lettuce and soy in your diet every day. A nice option for a meal could be a salad with these items, including soy cheese.

17. One way to reduce the appearance of cellulite is to tone up your body with some light to moderate weight training. Weight training will build the underlying muscle structure and make skin appear more taunt and smooth. Start with small weights of 1-3 pounds to avoid injury. Light to medium level weight training can help reduce unsightly cellulite. Give it a try!

18. Try using your hands to knead the areas of your body affected by cellulite problems. This may sound weird, but in fact that kneading helps circulate blood through your body. This, in turn, helps your body break down all of those ugly fat deposits that you are worrying over.

19. Try wearing "Tonewalker" sandals to fight that cellulite. These sandals actually are designed to

help make your muscles work a lot harder while walking. This in turn firms your muscles and combats that unsightly cellulite! It's an amazing benefit. Just think - every step that you take will actually help you combat those areas.

20. Dehydration is not your friend, and it certainly does you no favors when it comes to cellulite. Get up each morning and reach for a glass of water. Carry a water bottle with you throughout the day so that you remember to continue drinking. And, stay away from things like coffee, which can have a dehydrating effect.

21. If you smoke, stop. Smoking only makes cellulite worse. Not only does smoking introduce toxins into your skin, it makes it tougher. This worsens cellulite. Wrinkles and aging signs also get worse. If stopping is hard for you, talk to your primary care physician about your options.

22. To reduce the appearance of cellulite, make sure you exercise on a regular basis. Make sure you work up a good sweat when you exercise. Sweating helps expel toxins from the body through the skin. Exercise also improves your body's appearance by toning and tightening, so you look better even if you have cellulite.

23. You can fight off cellulite by using creams and products that contain caffeine. You can not get the same results by drinking a lot of coffee or other beverages that have caffeine. Using caffeinated beauty products can keep skin tighter for hours. The caffeine in them works by temporarily eliminating the connective tissue's water. This makes any dents in the skin less noticeable.

24. Don't stress too much. Stress is a big contributor to cellulite. Stress results in excess cortisol, which tends to boost fat storage while also thinning out the skin. Try yoga or meditation. Go for long, relaxing walks. Find something that is calming and will work best for you, then get enough sleep nightly.

25. Consider adding Murad's Firming and Toning serum to your beauty regime. It doesn't just have caffeine, but also includes a few more ingredients which make it a one-two punch for skin care. It has cayenne, for example, which helps to stimulate the skin's blood flow, improving its look and quality.

26. Add more fatty acids to your diet in order to reduce cellulite. They help to make connective tissue around your fat cells stronger. Also, they

help to slow down the production of fat cells, thus reducing cellulite. Good sources of fatty acids include blackcurrent seed oil, olive oil, fish oil, and flackseed oil.

27. Go out for a walk each day. Getting more exercise daily will help you avoid cellulite and can help eliminate what is already there. You will not need to join a gym or start running hundreds of miles each week to benefit. Just a nice walk each day is enough to help reduce the effects of cellulite.

28. Smoking can contribute to cellulite. It is a known fact that smoking speeds up the aging process. The faster you age, the more likely you are to begin seeing cellulite form. If you quit, your skin will become thicker, your body will become healthier and you will be able to battle your cellulite more effectively.

29. Use moisturizer daily. While moisturizer won't all of a sudden cure you from cellulite, what it will do is plump up your skin and make it look healthier. It'll hydrate you, and that leads to less of that cellulite being seen when you are out in public. Try moisturizing twice a day, once right after a shower.

30. You likely have tried a firming cream before, and while it might not give the best results alone, using it in conjunction with the other tips you read here will give you the boost you need to look your best. Estee Lauder provides the best option in their Body Performance line.

31. Use a body brush on your cellulite. This will help rid your skin of dead cells. It boosts lymphatic flow and works to stimulate your circulation. This encourages skin cell draining. Skin cell draining can result in less cellulite. Try this procedure two times a day using straight long strokes for the best results.

32. Want to quickly get all eyes away from your cellulite? Brush a shiny bronzer up and down the front of your legs where they are tight and cellulite-free. This will draw the eye to the front of your body and away from your problem areas, ensuring only the best of you is shown off.

33. Applying lotion to areas in which you have cellulite can help get rid of it. By rubbing lotion on your areas of cellulite in a circular motion, you are promoting circulation and reducing fatty deposits. These two factor put together can help you greatly reduce the appearance of cellulite on your skin.

34. Add a little dance to your life. It sounds like fun, and it's great for battling cellulite too! Dance can have a large amount of cardio exercise built right into it, and that's important for beating that bothersome cellulite. Plus, it's something that you can get your family involved with as well.

35. If you need help when you're trying to get rid of cellulite, you may want to try cardiovascular exercise. If you regularly exercise and try targeting areas with cellulite, you can beat it. Try running or bike riding to help rid your thighs and behind of that unsightly, unwanted cellulite.

36. If you are looking to get rid of cellulite, you should focus on eating a balanced diet on a regular basis. Numerous studies have shown that yo-yo dieting leaves most people with excess fatty deposits in the hips, thighs and rear. Try finding a solid, healthy diet and sticking to it.

37. If you have a lot of stress in your life, it is crucial that you do what you can to relax. Stress causes a myriad of problems in the body, not the least of which is the fact that it can keep you from producing healthy skin. Try going for an evening walk or setting aside a few minutes each day to take a warm bath.

38. If you have cellulite in your mid-abdominal region, try doing some crunches. Each crunch will force your abdominal muscles to tighten up work hard. The fat in that area is used to provide energy to this work out. What you will get is less fat your abdominal region and a more toned mid-section.

39. If you have cellulite in your thigh region, you should get into cycling. Go for a long bike ride a few times a week. When your legs pump the pedals, your thigh muscles work and burn off the fat in that region. You will notice that your thighs will begin to look leaner and firmer.

40. Add more fatty acids to your diet in order to reduce cellulite. They help to make connective tissue around your fat cells stronger. Also, they help to slow down the production of fat cells, thus reducing cellulite. Good sources of fatty acids include blackcurrent seed oil, olive oil, fish oil, and flackseed oil.

41. Go out for a walk each day. Getting more exercise daily will help you avoid cellulite and can help eliminate what is already there. You will not need to join a gym or start running hundreds of miles each week to benefit. Just a nice walk each

day is enough to help reduce the effects of cellulite.

42. Drink enough clean water. This will help you to flush toxins and extra sodium in your system. When you have extra sodium in your body and retain water, that can eventually cause cellulite. Drinking enough water will help you to avoid those dimples. If you don't like water, you can flavor it as well.

43. To give the illusion of smoother skin, put on a self-tanning lotion first where the bumps are. After that, spray yourself with another self-tanning product which gives you full coverage. This will make the bumps disappear while giving you a slimming tan that makes your whole body look its best.

44. Try some lifestyle changes to prevent or reduce cellulite. While a lot of therapies or options that are cosmetic can be used against cellulite, not a lot of evidence is out there to prove that it works. Follow a sound diet plan and work out often to keep hormones in balance. Avoid situations that cause hormones to get out of balance, such as stress.

45. If you're self conscious about your cellulite while working out, try wearing shorts that are made to make your legs and buttocks appear slimmer. Some shorts even contain caffeine and enzymes that are included to reduce the appearance of dimpling once you are doing working out and take off the shorts.

46. So, you want to get rid of your cellulite and you are thinking about sinking a ton of money having your problem areas liposuctioned. Yes, liposuction is a surgical procedure which removes fat. However, it removes deep fat, not the cellulite fat which is just below the skin's surface. In some cases, liposuction actually creates more dimpling of the skin and worsen the appearance of your cellulite.

47. Cellulite is caused by fat deposits under the skin, typically located on the thighs and buttocks at puberty. Many women and some men who tend to be somewhat overweight have a considerable amount of cellulite. The most effective way to get rid of it is to lose the excess weight.

48. Because cellulite is made of fat, you can reduce your fat percentage by eating healthier foods and drinking more water. If you already do these things, try massaging the areas to help break up

the fat under your skin. Cellulite is hereditary and also very stubborn, so there's no instant cure.

49. If cellulite has you mentally down, remember that it's something that many people battle. This isn't just you. Cellulite affects millions of people, from friends to celebrities, from family to royalty. There's no reason to let it get the best of you mentally. Keep your chin up and work towards beating it.

50. Avoid tight fitting underwear. Underwear that has tight elastic across the buttocks, should be avoided. Blood flow to these regions will be impaired. This limited flow of blood can add to the formation of cellulite. Occasionally wearing this underwear is fine, but continuous wear will most likely lead to increased cellulite.

51. Try to stay away from dairy products which are full fat. These items have tons of saturated fat which the body can't break down and use very easily. Instead, it will store it and turn it into more cellulite. Stick to no-fat and low-fat options when it comes to dairy.

52. If you have cellulite that you have been trying to get rid of, you should try getting more exercise. While this will not make the cellulite go away, it

will redistribute some of the fatty deposits and remove some of the excess fluids. This will make the problem areas look a lot smoother.

53. Do not believe the myth that cardio is the best way to get rid of cellulite. While it does work to some degree, you have to combine it with other exercises. This will not totally remove any cellulite in the body, but it will definitely improve the way it looks.

54. Try bursts of intensive exercise to lower those cellulite fat deposits. A good exercise to do this with is jumping rope. Keep the exercise short and intense helps target those areas you are having trouble with, while not disrupting your day. Try to find a few minutes every few hours and get a few repetitions in.

55. Drink lots of water. This is the easiest and really most effective thing that you can do to battle cellulite. If you get eight glasses per day into your diet, that water will help get toxins out of your body. Plus it'll pump up your circulation too. All of which will lead to less cellulite.

56. If you have cellulite and want to diminish its appearance, try brushing and massaging your skin. Brushing and massaging your skin

stimulates your lymphatic system and helps eliminate toxins from your body. Use a skin brush to target specific areas where you have cellulite. Brush skin in circular motions a few times a week to help break down fatty deposits responsible for the dimpled appearance.

57. Stay hydrated and consume foods that contain healthy oils. Maybe you're not sure why you should do this. When you keep your body hydrated, you eliminate a lot of the dimpling look you get with cellulite. When you are properly hydrated, your skin is plumped up so dimples aren't readily apparent. It's an effective and easy way to fight it.

58. If you have cellulite in your mid-abdominal region, try doing some crunches. Each crunch will force your abdominal muscles to tighten up work hard. The fat in that area is used to provide energy to this work out. What you will get is less fat your abdominal region and a more toned mid-section.

59. Because cellulite normally appears on the thighs, legs, and buttocks, try toning these areas. Lunges and squats are easy exercises you can do anywhere to strengthen these areas. Building up the muscle can help to alleviate the appearance

of the fat deposits that can appear underneath the skin to create cellulite.

60. Drink copious amounts of water to beat cellulite. If you drink more water, your skin will look better. Hydration flushes toxins from the body while keeping everything wrinkle-free and taut. This allows your entire skin to look aan feel great, thus keeping cellulite from occurring.

61. Lower your stress levels. You may be unaware of this, but stress changes the hormone balance in your body. This may contribute to your body's ability to shed itself of unwanted fat. You will be much slimmer when you are less stressed.

62. To reduce the toxins that worsen the appearance of cellulite, give your trouble areas a massage everyday. You can use massage tools, brushes, or even specially shaped soaps to give yourself the massage. The massage will stimulate your circulatory and lymphatic systems which will help move toxins out of the areas you target.

63. Use moisturizer daily. While moisturizer won't all of a sudden cure you from cellulite, what it will do is plump up your skin and make it look healthier. It'll hydrate you, and that leads to less of that cellulite being seen when you are out in

public. Try moisturizing twice a day, once right after a shower.

64. Get more protein into your daily diet. A big issue that affects cellulite is water retention. That's something that protein can really help with as protein actually helps absorb a lot of that fluid that's just sitting around. Try to eat at least three portions of healthy protein every single day.

65. If using squats to combat cellulite, be sure you are doing them at least three times per week. You should be doing at least fifteen squats per workout to ensure the best results. If you can do more, go for it! The tighter your legs are, the leaner they will look.

66. So, you want to get rid of your cellulite and you are thinking about sinking a ton of money having your problem areas liposuctioned. Yes, liposuction is a surgical procedure which removes fat. However, it removes deep fat, not the cellulite fat which is just below the skin's surface. In some cases, liposuction actually creates more dimpling of the skin and worsen the appearance of your cellulite.

67. To address your cellulite problem, eat foods that are make your skin cells stronger. Extra cellulite makes your skin look bumpy and uneven. Foods high in lecithin strengthen your skin cells and are effective in getting rid of extra cellulite. Include in your diet plenty of apples, spinach, cauliflower, eggs, and soy.

68. Reducing stress can help reduce cellulite. Stress causes you hormones to be affected. Then your body starts producing stress hormones like cortisol which can affect your appetite and the way that your body metabolizes things. So try to keep stress at a manageable level and have ways to deal with it when it does appear.

69. The gym offers many ways for you to exercise, but focus on the cardio machines if your goal is to beat cellulite. For example, running on a treadmill, biking on a recumbent bicycle or even hitting the elliptical can get your heart pumping. The harder you work, the more fat you will shed.

70. Try using a sculpting or firming gel. Applying sculpting or firming gel to your problem areas can tighten them up and cut down on ugly cellulite. Try applying these products after you get out of the shower. By applying them after a

shower, your skin will be able to absorb them more deeply.

71. You can remove cellulite from your body by eating a healthy diet. Eating many fruits and vegetables can help. The alkaline ash they create is important to the process. Juicing is a fantastic way to get your body all the vegetables and fruits it needs.

72. If you are looking to get rid of cellulite, you should focus on eating a balanced diet on a regular basis. Numerous studies have shown that yo-yo dieting leaves most people with excess fatty deposits in the hips, thighs and rear. Try finding a solid, healthy diet and sticking to it.

73. Pick up a cellulite mitt and work on your troubled areas from right inside your home. Cellulite mitts have raised ridges and knobs that help promote circulation and blood flow when you scrub your body with them. This then helps your body break down those pockets of ugly cellulite.

74. A natural way to get rid of cellulite is by switching your salt. Believe it or not, table salt could be causing you to have cellulite; its acidity depletes you of minerals you need in your body.

It makes your body more "toxic." Switch over to Himalayan crystal salt or Celtic sea salt.

75. Get daily exercise into your life. Burning fat is essential if you're looking to rid yourself of cellulite. Obviously, if you don't exercise, you'll be more prone to cellulite occurring. Just 30 minutes of high impact exercise a day can make a real difference to how you look. It's worth it.

76. If you have cellulite and you are a smoker, it is time for you to quit. Smoking reduces the food supply to your skin and puts more harmful toxins in your body. This damages the elasticity of your skin, making it more prone to cellulite. If you did not have enough of a reason to quit smoking before, you do now.

77. If you're a smoker, stop the habit now. You may not realize it, but that smoking is increasing your issues with cellulite as it adds toxins into your body and affects your skin's supply of food. Your skin will respond very kindly to you dropping this habit. Over time, you'll see a lot less cellulite.

78. Since cellulite can be caused by wearing tight fitting garments around the waist and lower body, it is best to wear clothing that does not

bind and reduce circulation. Some people wear compression garments to minimize the lumpy appearance of the condition. This may minimize the bumpy appearance, but does not correct the problem.

79. Get more protein into your daily diet. A big issue that affects cellulite is water retention. That's something that protein can really help with as protein actually helps absorb a lot of that fluid that's just sitting around. Try to eat at least three portions of healthy protein every single day.

80. Try specialized serums that are formulated to reduce cellulite; they can often reduce the number of dimples on your skin. If the product you are considering has caffeine in it, this can help you to see a difference within a fortnight. Nivea is one such company with products like this.

81. Both overweight and thin people can get cellulite. However, gaining weight can attribute to cellulite. So, losing weight also means losing the cellulite. The most effective way to lose both weight and cellulite is by doing resistance training on your butt and legs and cardiovascular

exercises. You may not see results overnight, but when you do see them, you will be pleased!

82. Work on eliminating bread for no less than 30 days if your cellulite is stubborn. Your body treats bread as a sugar, and will increase your chances of having cellulite. Try getting it out of your diet completely, and then check to see if it has helped to reduce the appearance of cellulite.

83. When it comes to combating any fat, cardio is your best friend. When you exercise, be it riding a bike, going for a swim or hitting the gym, you're burning fat. The more fat you burn, the tighter your body will become. To get rid of cellulite, boost your heart rate!

84. Want to burn away your cellulite? Go for a walk after dinner. Studies show that a walk within 20 minutes of dinner helps your blood sugar stay stable and makes it so that you don't pack on as many pounds. On top of that, a brisk walk will burn fat you already have.

85. Looking to slim down your body and get rid of cellulite? Consider playing a sport. The harder you work, the more fat you burn, and that is exactly what cellulite is made of. If you don't

have any fat, you won't have cellulite either, so go join a team and have fun!

86. If all other solutions fail, you may want to consider liposuction to battle cellulite. This is an serious medical treatment, so it should not be the first thing you go to. And it's not foolproof, as some cellulite can actually look worse after liposuction. Weigh your options carefully and talk with your doctor.

87. Try using your hands to knead the areas of your body affected by cellulite problems. This may sound weird, but in fact that kneading helps circulate blood through your body. This, in turn, helps your body break down all of those ugly fat deposits that you are worrying over.

88. Make moisturizing a part of your daily skin routine. There are many reasons why you should do this. It can make it easier to take on your cellulite for one. When applying lotion, massage your problematic areas daily. This will break down some fatty deposits which also fights cellulite.

89. Drinking a lot of water will help improve the appearance of cellulite on the body, so make sure to consume as much as you can. Some people

say this is because drinking water removes harmful toxins that cause cellulite. The truth is that it improves skin elasticity, so the skin around the cellulite will look tighter and smoother.

90. In order to reduce cellulite, you should drink plenty of water. Water helps flush your body of toxins which accumulate in your body and create cellulite. Water also keeps your skin hydrated, giving a smoother appearance to your skin. Avoid drinks like coffee, tea and alcohol which can dehydrate you.

91. Diet may just be the key to losing your cellulite. Consume more veggies and fruits. They leave behind an alkaline ash that will help you to start looking your best. Juicing is another way to help improve your skin.

92. Increasing your activity level can be a big help in the fight against cellulite. Cardio classes, strength training and even brisk walking all help to burn the fat that goes into making that ugly cellulite on your thighs. Increase exercises that tone your thighs to keep your skin elastic and smooth.

93. You can fight off cellulite by using creams and products that contain caffeine. You can not get the same results by drinking a lot of coffee or

other beverages that have caffeine. Using caffeinated beauty products can keep skin tighter for hours. The caffeine in them works by temporarily eliminating the connective tissue's water. This makes any dents in the skin less noticeable.

94. To help minimize the appearance of cellulite on the skin, consider taking action to improve the circulation in the affected areas. By massaging the skin vigorously with a hand or with an electric massage tool, it is possible to accomplish this goal with ease. The bumpy look of the cellulite will soon be far less noticeable.

95. Use a moisturizer. However, try not to fall victim to claims of miracle results. There is no one product that is going to get rid of all your cellulite, all on its own. Still, a moisturizer is important, and you should try and select something that was designed to target cellulite.

96. To reduce the toxins that worsen the appearance of cellulite, give your trouble areas a massage everyday. You can use massage tools, brushes, or even specially shaped soaps to give yourself the massage. The massage will stimulate your circulatory and lymphatic systems which will help move toxins out of the areas you target.

97. Despite claims made by different products, there's no way to magically get rid of cellulite in a short amount of time. However, you can camouflage your cellulite. On darker skin tones, cellulite is less noticeable. If your skin is light-toned, apply a self-tanner before going to the beach or pool in your new bathing suit. The dimpling of your skin won't be so noticeable.

98. Go out for a walk each day. Getting more exercise daily will help you avoid cellulite and can help eliminate what is already there. You will not need to join a gym or start running hundreds of miles each week to benefit. Just a nice walk each day is enough to help reduce the effects of cellulite.

99. Use moisturizer daily. While moisturizer won't all of a sudden cure you from cellulite, what it will do is plump up your skin and make it look healthier. It'll hydrate you, and that leads to less of that cellulite being seen when you are out in public. Try moisturizing twice a day, once right after a shower.

100. To prevent cellulite from forming, eat a diet that is low in fat and sugar. Cellulite develops when your body produces too much fat. When

you eat a low-fat, low-sugar diet, you keep your weight down and your body muscles toned. Eat more fruits and vegetables instead for a leaner looking body.

101.   Try moisturizing and massaging your skin to fight off cellulite. Skin needs an extra hand from time to time. Help it by moisturizing it. Then, break down its fatty cells via kneading in the areas that are prone to cellulite. Combining these two methods tens to be effective. To boost results, apply moisturizer in a circular motion to boost circulation and cut down on fatty deposits.

102.   Change some of your habits to rid yourself of cellulite. You can get rid of cellulite through therapy and cosmetic surgery, but evidence shows this may not work. Just exercise and have a good diet that helps you maintain hormone levels that are normal. Avoid situations that cause hormones to get out of balance, such as stress.

103.   So, you want to get rid of your cellulite and you are thinking about sinking a ton of money having your problem areas liposuctioned. Yes, liposuction is a surgical procedure which removes fat. However, it removes deep fat, not the cellulite fat which is just below the skin's

surface. In some cases, liposuction actually creates more dimpling of the skin and worsen the appearance of your cellulite.

104.   Regular use of moisturizing lotion is recommended. It is ideal to keep the skin properly hydrated with moisturizer. It can really help you battle cellulite. Make sure that you massage the areas upon application. Massaging it into your skin will break up fatty deposits, cutting down on cellulite as well.

105.   Try using a sculpting or firming gel. Applying sculpting or firming gel to your problem areas can tighten them up and cut down on ugly cellulite. Try applying these products after you get out of the shower. By applying them after a shower, your skin will be able to absorb them more deeply.

106.   In order to reduce cellulite, you should drink plenty of water. Water helps flush your body of toxins which accumulate in your body and create cellulite. Water also keeps your skin hydrated, giving a smoother appearance to your skin. Avoid drinks like coffee, tea and alcohol which can dehydrate you.

107.   Cut down on the salt that you eat in your diet. Salt may taste good, but it actually makes you retain fluids. This can be very problematic and increase cellulite pockets. If you lower the amount of salt you eat, you could see a surprising amount of improvement quite quickly.

108.   One great way to get rid of cellulite is to lose excess fat that your body is carrying. Fat loss techniques vary, but one tried and true method is to take up a low carbohydrate diet. By increasing your intake of protein and fat and decreasing your carbohydrates, you can successfully burn off some of your stored fat and thus reduce cellulite formation.

109.   To keep cellulite at bay, try maintaining a regular exercise regimen that includes lunges. These particular moves really help firm up the thighs. These exercise build up lean muscle in the thighs and buttocks, which cellulite is generally present. Maintain proper form when doing these exercises to keep away the cellulite by not letting your knees go too far over your toes. Also, keep the heel on the front foot pressed into the floor while squeezing your glutes.

110.   Since cellulite can be caused by wearing tight fitting garments around the waist and lower

body, it is best to wear clothing that does not bind and reduce circulation. Some people wear compression garments to minimize the lumpy appearance of the condition. This may minimize the bumpy appearance, but does not correct the problem.

111.   If you have got problems with cellulite, consider cutting down on your daily sugar intake. Sugar is a primary cause of cellulite, because it creates a build up of fat in your body. This leaves you with those unsightly dimples that are so difficult to get rid of! Cut down on sugar and loose cellulite.

112.   Because cellulite normally appears on the thighs, legs, and buttocks, try toning these areas. Lunges and squats are easy exercises you can do anywhere to strengthen these areas. Building up the muscle can help to alleviate the appearance of the fat deposits that can appear underneath the skin to create cellulite.

113.   Remember that cellulite is not a condemnation; cellulite does not indicate being overweight or unhealthy. Many women deal with cellulite, and unfortunately it is not something that is easily removed. Do not let your self

esteem falter just because you have what most other women also have.

114.   You can try using bronzer to fight off your cellulite. A faux tan in the area that are prone to tan make your skin look better and draw attention away from the dimples. The darker colors can make these dimples appear smaller. Just make sure to exfoliate first with a gentle body scrub on those areas, then you can use a tanning lotion or spray.

115.   Cellulite is often the result of accumulated toxins within the body. Therefore, to really start eliminating the condition and the bumpy appearance everyone dreads, embark on a clean diet of unprocessed foods and fresh water. It will not be long at all until the cellulite starts to become a distant memory.

116.   Poor blood circulation could be a contributing factor to your cellulite. Avoid sitting for extended periods of time. If you must sit for work, try to get up at least every half hour for five minutes or so. That will get the blood flowing and will reduce the effects that cellulite has on your buttocks and upper thighs.

117.   To give the illusion of smoother skin, put on a self-tanning lotion first where the bumps are. After that, spray yourself with another self-tanning product which gives you full coverage. This will make the bumps disappear while giving you a slimming tan that makes your whole body look its best.

118.   Find ways to relieve high stress. High levels of stress can boost your catecholamines adrenalin. This hormone has been found to help evolve cellulite. Find ways to remove stress from your environment or lifestyle. Meditation can help to reduce stress in places such as work or home. Try walking or jogging, when time permits, to reduce stress as well.

119.   To improve the appearance of cellulite, use a good anti-cellulite cream that has phosphodiesterase inhibitors listed as part of the ingredients. With daily use you should see a decrease in the dimpling that accompanies cellulite. You can realistically expect to see the difference after about 6 weeks of continuous use.

120.   Ask your partner for a massage. Or you can look to get professional massages instead. While that sounds great alone, it also has major benefits to battling cellulite as well. That massage helps

stimulate blood flowing throughout the area. That blood flow can help you combat those pockets of cellulite.

121.   Brush your skin with a body brush. The body brush helps your skin in multiple ways. It removes dead skin, boots your overall circulation, and even improves what's called lymphatic flow. That in fact helps lower the amount of cellulite that you are dealing with. Make it a habit to brush at least twice per day.

122.   Try using a body brush on your skin. Brushing your skin with a body brush is a great way to reduce cellulite. It removes dead skin cells and stimulates blood flow. Brush your problem areas in an upward direction to break up fatty deposits and cut down on some of that unsightly cellulite.

123.   Do not buy any creams that promise to help you get rid of cellulite because these things never work. The only things these products may offer is a temporary reprieve. You should keep your money in your pocket because any who offers a miracle cure is out to scam you.

124.   Cellulite may be caused by poor diet choices that are high in fat, salt, carbohydrates and

minimal fiber. People who smoke, do not exercise enough and sit or stand for extended periods of time are also more likely to develop cellulite. Genetics may also make some people predisposed to the condition.

125.   If you're a smoker, stop the habit now. You may not realize it, but that smoking is increasing your issues with cellulite as it adds toxins into your body and affects your skin's supply of food. Your skin will respond very kindly to you dropping this habit. Over time, you'll see a lot less cellulite.

126.   To reduce the toxins that worsen the appearance of cellulite, give your trouble areas a massage everyday. You can use massage tools, brushes, or even specially shaped soaps to give yourself the massage. The massage will stimulate your circulatory and lymphatic systems which will help move toxins out of the areas you target.

127.   It is possible to disguise cellulite with a good tan. Even though this will not make cellulite disappear, it becomes less noticeable to the eye. Although exposing yourself to the sun is not ideal, you can substitute that with a self-tanner or spray tan lotion. Always be smart and aware about which brand you use.

128.   Get more protein into your daily diet. A big issue that affects cellulite is water retention. That's something that protein can really help with as protein actually helps absorb a lot of that fluid that's just sitting around. Try to eat at least three portions of healthy protein every single day.

129.   Both overweight and thin people can get cellulite. However, gaining weight can attribute to cellulite. So, losing weight also means losing the cellulite. The most effective way to lose both weight and cellulite is by doing resistance training on your butt and legs and cardiovascular exercises. You may not see results overnight, but when you do see them, you will be pleased!

130.   Try using a self tanner to hide that cellulite. If you are starting to battle cellulite but still want a way to hide what's there currently, a self tanning cream can really do wonders. The cream helps even out skin tone, which, in effect, helps hide that cellulite from view.

131.   When it comes to combating any fat, cardio is your best friend. When you exercise, be it riding a bike, going for a swim or hitting the gym, you're burning fat. The more fat you burn,

the tighter your body will become. To get rid of cellulite, boost your heart rate!

132.   Because cellulite is made of fat, you can reduce your fat percentage by eating healthier foods and drinking more water. If you already do these things, try massaging the areas to help break up the fat under your skin. Cellulite is hereditary and also very stubborn, so there's no instant cure.

133.   Alternate your showers between hot and cold. When you're showering, try switching to cool water for a few minutes and then back to hot. Go back and forth a few times as you shower. This can really do wonders for the circulation in your skin, which can help get rid of cellulite.

134.   Every bit of exercise you do will help, so try to avoid the lazy man's way out. For example, take the stairs instead of an elevator or escalator. Park at the back of the mall lot and go for a long stroll. The more you do, the smoother your body will be.

135.   To reduce your cellulite, you need to get a handle on the stress in your life. Stress can cause hormonal changes that may affect your skin.

Cortisol is a type of stress hormone that may cause skin thinning and increased fat storage. It may also slow growth hormone production that helps create healthy skin. Try relaxing by doing things like cycling, yoga, walking, and the like. Also, make sure you get plenty of sleep.

136.   A soothing massage can be a fantastic way to minimize your cellulite! The kneading action is great for circulation, and can improve the strength and function of the connective tissues right below the skin's surface. Just one more reason to make an appointment at your favorite spa for a fantastic massage!

137.   Obviously, eating junk food will only make your cellulite worse. If you must, treat yourself to one item per week, but otherwise, avoid it like the plague. The worse the food you eat, the worse you will look and you will end up derailing all of your hard work beating cellulite.

138.   If you have cellulite that you have been trying to get rid of, you should try getting more exercise. While this will not make the cellulite go away, it will redistribute some of the fatty deposits and remove some of the excess fluids. This will make the problem areas look a lot smoother.

139.   Drinking water is the key to getting rid of cellulite. Staying hydrated may not cure cellulite, but it can stop it from occurring or reoccurring. It works to maintain proper skin hydration. It also flushes out the toxins that may cause cellulite. Drink at least six glasses of water a day.

140.   Try bursts of intensive exercise to lower those cellulite fat deposits. A good exercise to do this with is jumping rope. Keep the exercise short and intense helps target those areas you are having trouble with, while not disrupting your day. Try to find a few minutes every few hours and get a few repetitions in.

141.   Plastic surgery has been one way that people have dealt with cellulite. However, this should be seen as your last resort. There are safer, cheaper ways to get rid of your cellulite. Surgery should only be used as a completely last resort.

142.   Exercising and losing weight can help reduce the appearance of cellulite. Because cellulite is just excess fat being stored near the surface of your skin, reducing the fat in your body can lead to a reduction in cellulite. Good cellulite eliminating exercises include running or jogging, swimming, and yoga or pilates.

143.   One of the best things you can do about cellulite is to watch what you eat. You need to eat a diet that has less processed foods and fats and more fiber, fruit and vegetables. Foods with chemicals preservatives and such are not able to be fully flushed from your body.

144.   Want to get rid of that pesky cellulite? Rub some coffee grounds into the area. Give it a good, deep massage and allow the coffee to exfoliate the top layers of skin. Add a little olive oil for lubrication and to ensure the coffee doesn't just fall off all over your floor.

145.   Make sure that you are exercising regularly. Aerobics, like dancing, running, or cycling, burns extra calories while toning your muscles. Remember that cellulite is stored fat, and exercising can help to get rid of this fat. Aerobics are also important for heart health and your general well-being, since it gets your heart pumping.

146.   Use a body brush on your cellulite. It will help remove dead skin cells. It also stimulates your circulation and will improve lymphatic flow. Skin cell draining ensues, and this can reduce the appearance of cellulite on your body. Attempt to

do this twice daily. Use longer strokes to see the best result.

147.   Both overweight and thin people can get cellulite. However, gaining weight can attribute to cellulite. So, losing weight also means losing the cellulite. The most effective way to lose both weight and cellulite is by doing resistance training on your butt and legs and cardiovascular exercises. You may not see results overnight, but when you do see them, you will be pleased!

148.   In the battle against cellulite, many people have found real success with the multiple formulations of topical treatment available on market. However, the key to getting lasting results lies within commitment and routine. When applied religiously on a daily basis, it is possible to see a change sooner than you may have thought possible.

149.   Use caffeine filled body scrubs on the areas of your body in which cellulite is a problem. These scrubs can help to break up any fatty deposits in the area causing you the problems. Look for an exfoliator that has caffeine, avocado oil and can be used generously in the area.

150. Since there are not many tricks to getting rid of cellulite, work on the skin itself as an alternative. Vitamins can be taken and you can drink water regularly so the skin has more elasticity which makes it smoother looking. Men have thicker epidermises, which is why cellulite doesn't occur as often with them.

151. Get a tan to reduce how visible your cellulite is. All things, even cellulite, will look smaller in a mirror if they are darker. It is important that you begin with skin exfoliation to help smooth the skin's surface by using a good body scrub, then apply the tanning lotion.

152. To stop cellulite from ever appearing, you need to get your protein. To create elastin and collagen, you need protein in your body. That doesn't mean you should start scarfing down some bacon! Enjoy lean meats, fish, nuts and no fat dairy products instead to ensure you don't pack on the pounds, too.

153. One way to reduce the appearance of cellulite is to tone up your body with some light to moderate weight training. Weight training will build the underlying muscle structure and make skin appear more taunt and smooth. Start with small weights of 1-3 pounds to avoid injury.

Light to medium level weight training can help reduce unsightly cellulite. Give it a try!

154.   There is little you can do to get rid of cellulite, since it is hereditary. Try wearing longer skirts or pants to cover these areas if you are very self conscious. Most women experience cellulite, and it does not mean you are unhealthy or that you need to lose weight.

155.   If you have cellulite that you have been trying to get rid of, you should try getting more exercise. While this will not make the cellulite go away, it will redistribute some of the fatty deposits and remove some of the excess fluids. This will make the problem areas look a lot smoother.

156.   Try using your hands to knead the areas of your body affected by cellulite problems. This may sound weird, but in fact that kneading helps circulate blood through your body. This, in turn, helps your body break down all of those ugly fat deposits that you are worrying over.

157.   If you drink tea, drink green tea. Green tea can break down some of the fatty deposits in your body. This obviously contributes to less

cellulite. Green tea capsules are an alternative option for you.

158.   A natural way to get rid of cellulite is by switching your salt. Believe it or not, table salt could be causing you to have cellulite; its acidity depletes you of minerals you need in your body. It makes your body more "toxic." Switch over to Himalayan crystal salt or Celtic sea salt.

159.   Plastic surgery can help eliminate cellulite, but it should just be used as the absolute last resort. It can be dangerous, though. Surgery should only be used if nothing else worked.

160.   Make sure to eat a healthy diet. It's important that your skin gets all the nutrients it needs. Foods rich in antioxidants will help produce collagen, which keeps your skin plump. Plenty of vitamin E, C, and omega-3 fatty acids will greatly improve the feel and texture of your skin.

161.   If you want to get rid of excess cellulite under your skin, bump up your exercise regimen in that particular area. When you focus your workout in a specific region, the fat in that area is used to fuel the workout. That will help tone up your muscles and firm up your skin.

162.   Make sure that you're drinking plenty of
water. There are many reasons to drink water.
When you're not drinking enough water, sodium
can build up. This can cause you to retain water,
producing excess cellulite. Drinking plenty of
water can remedy this and keep your skin
hydrated, cutting down on cellulite.

163.   Hormones are key to cellulite formation,
which means having your levels checked. Insulin,
adrenal hormones, prolactin and hormones
produced by the thyroid all act to produce
cellulite. Estrogen may be a major factor
involved as well, though studies are still being
done to determine its full impact. Abnormal
levels in any of these hormones could be a cause
of your cellulite.

164.   Use a moisturizer. However, try not to fall
victim to claims of miracle results. There is no
one product that is going to get rid of all your
cellulite, all on its own. Still, a moisturizer is
important, and you should try and select
something that was designed to target cellulite.

165.   To reduce cellulite, reduce your everyday
stress level. Most folks don't know this, but
hormone levels are heavily impacted by stress.
When your hormonal balance is off, it can cause

your body to store more fat. Reducing stress will lead to a healthier, better-looking you.

166.   To reduce the toxins that worsen the appearance of cellulite, give your trouble areas a massage everyday. You can use massage tools, brushes, or even specially shaped soaps to give yourself the massage. The massage will stimulate your circulatory and lymphatic systems which will help move toxins out of the areas you target.

167.   Despite claims made by different products, there's no way to magically get rid of cellulite in a short amount of time. However, you can camouflage your cellulite. On darker skin tones, cellulite is less noticeable. If your skin is light-toned, apply a self-tanner before going to the beach or pool in your new bathing suit. The dimpling of your skin won't be so noticeable.

168.   Use moisturizer daily. While moisturizer won't all of a sudden cure you from cellulite, what it will do is plump up your skin and make it look healthier. It'll hydrate you, and that leads to less of that cellulite being seen when you are out in public. Try moisturizing twice a day, once right after a shower.

169.   You likely have tried a firming cream before, and while it might not give the best results alone, using it in conjunction with the other tips you read here will give you the boost you need to look your best. Estee Lauder provides the best option in their Body Performance line.

170.   If you want a temporary quick-fix to reducing you cellulite, apply a caffeine-based cream to your skin. Caffeine temporarily gets rid of water in the connective tissues, reducing the dimple appearance in the skin. Before applying the cream, make sure you exfoliate with a body scrub or loofah to maximize the effects of the cream.

171.   When looking at your cellulite problem, it is important to know if you have a genetic predisposition. Gender plays the major part; however, factors such as race, metabolic rate and circulatory issues are involved as well. Being genetically susceptible to cellulite will have an impact on your approach to prevention.

172.   To stop cellulite from ever appearing, you need to get your protein. To create elastin and collagen, you need protein in your body. That doesn't mean you should start scarfing down some bacon! Enjoy lean meats, fish, nuts and no

fat dairy products instead to ensure you don't pack on the pounds, too.

173.   Do not buy any creams that promise to help you get rid of cellulite because these things never work. The only things these products may offer is a temporary reprieve. You should keep your money in your pocket because any who offers a miracle cure is out to scam you.

174.   Cellulite can be mitigated to a large degree by staying hydrated. Staying hydrated may not cure cellulite, but it can stop it from occurring or reoccurring. It works to maintain proper skin hydration. Water will also flush out toxins that can cause cellulite. Try drinking no fewer than six glasses daily.

175.   Eating healthy can reduce the presence of cellulite. Eating high-fiber foods and whole grains helps to remove toxins that increase cellulite. In addition, you can remove even more toxins with lots of water.

176.   Increasing your activity level can be a big help in the fight against cellulite. Cardio classes, strength training and even brisk walking all help to burn the fat that goes into making that ugly cellulite on your thighs. Increase exercises that

tone your thighs to keep your skin elastic and smooth.

177.   Make sure that you're drinking plenty of water. There are many reasons to drink water. When you're not drinking enough water, sodium can build up. This can cause you to retain water, producing excess cellulite. Drinking plenty of water can remedy this and keep your skin hydrated, cutting down on cellulite.

178.   Drink enough clean water. This will help you to flush toxins and extra sodium in your system. When you have extra sodium in your body and retain water, that can eventually cause cellulite. Drinking enough water will help you to avoid those dimples. If you don't like water, you can flavor it as well.

179.   Treat cellulite with a body brush. A body brush is useful in clearing out skins cells that are dead. It can also stimulate circulation and boost lymphatic flow. This process will allow your skin cells to drain, which can mitigate the effects of cellulite. Long strokes twice daily will give you the best results.

180.   Get more protein into your daily diet. A big issue that affects cellulite is water retention.

That's something that protein can really help with as protein actually helps absorb a lot of that fluid that's just sitting around. Try to eat at least three portions of healthy protein every single day.

181.   Find ways to relieve high stress. High levels of stress can boost your catecholamines adrenalin. This hormone has been found to help evolve cellulite. Find ways to remove stress from your environment or lifestyle. Meditation can help to reduce stress in places such as work or home. Try walking or jogging, when time permits, to reduce stress as well.

182.   If you massage your cellulite areas with an exfoliating scrub or knobbed massager, it can help to break up the fat areas and distribute it more evenly. If you use soaps or scrubs containing caffeine, it can help tighten your skin and reduce the appearance of lumps at the same time.

183.   You can help banish cellulite by not smoking. Smoking introduces toxins into your body. Those toxins interfere with your ability to easily flush your body and reduce the blood flow to areas of your body. Smoking also adds

wrinkles to your face so it is something that you should never do anyway.

184.   Apply cellulite-busting serum to your skin, which can reduce dimples and give your body a glowing appearance. Such products often contain caffeine and can make a difference in appearance in just a few short weeks. Nivea and various other companies sell products like this.

185.   To cut down cellulite, concentrate on lifestyle changes. While many therapies or cosmetic options are available to handle cellulite, not enough evidence exists to support their efficacy. Make sure that you eat well and get enough exercise. Avoiding stress is also very important for keeping your hormones in check.

186.   Massaging your cellulite with exfoliating scrubs or a massager with knobs can break up the fat and distribute it more evenly. You can also try using self tanner or serums made to make your skin look smoother. There is no magical formula for busting cellulite, but these can certainly help.

187.   Since you can't do much to eradicate your cellulite, focus on skin. When you take vitamins and drink water regularly, this can actually

improve the skin's elasticity which can make it appear smoother. The reason men have less cellulite is because their epidermis is thicker.

188.   One way to reduce the appearance of cellulite is to tone up your body with some light to moderate weight training. Weight training will build the underlying muscle structure and make skin appear more taunt and smooth. Start with small weights of 1-3 pounds to avoid injury. Light to medium level weight training can help reduce unsightly cellulite. Give it a try!

189.   Try to stay away from dairy products which are full fat. These items have tons of saturated fat which the body can't break down and use very easily. Instead, it will store it and turn it into more cellulite. Stick to no-fat and low-fat options when it comes to dairy.

190.   Did you know that by following a healthy diet plan, you may be able to reduce your cellulite? The first thing you need to trim is the amount of sugar that you use. Your fat cells absorb sugars, which causes them to expand. Next, you need to reduce your intake of salt. The sodium in the salt causes your body to retain water, which will also cause your cellulite to look worse.

191.   Brush your skin with a body brush. The body brush helps your skin in multiple ways. It removes dead skin, boots your overall circulation, and even improves what's called lymphatic flow. That in fact helps lower the amount of cellulite that you are dealing with. Make it a habit to brush at least twice per day.

192.   Green tea is also great to drink when you are trying to get rid of cellulite. Green tea is full of great ingredients that break down fat. This translates into less cellulite on your body. If you prefer, you can also buy green tea capsules that can be even more potent!

193.   One great way to get rid of cellulite is to lose excess fat that your body is carrying. Fat loss techniques vary, but one tried and true method is to take up a low carbohydrate diet. By increasing your intake of protein and fat and decreasing your carbohydrates, you can successfully burn off some of your stored fat and thus reduce cellulite formation.

194.   To reduce the appearance of cellulite, make sure you exercise on a regular basis. Make sure you work up a good sweat when you exercise. Sweating helps expel toxins from the body

through the skin. Exercise also improves your body's appearance by toning and tightening, so you look better even if you have cellulite.

195.   If you want to get rid of excess cellulite under your skin, bump up your exercise regimen in that particular area. When you focus your workout in a specific region, the fat in that area is used to fuel the workout. That will help tone up your muscles and firm up your skin.

196.   Some methods that have been used to remove cellulite include heat therapy, pneumatic massages, ultrasound and electrical stimulation. Unfortunately, none of these methods have been proven to work. Probably the most effective way to get rid of cellulite is to eat nutritious, low fat foods that are high in fiber. This causes weight loss and reduction of fat.

197.   Increasing your activity level can be a big help in the fight against cellulite. Cardio classes, strength training and even brisk walking all help to burn the fat that goes into making that ugly cellulite on your thighs. Increase exercises that tone your thighs to keep your skin elastic and smooth.

198.   It doesn't seem like it, but stress can actually be a cause of cellulite and other disorders. When a stressful situation occurs, the hormone Cortisol is let loose in your body. This is a hormone that boosts fat storage and thins out skin. Meditation and yoga are both great things to do if you're dealing with stress.

199.   Hormones are key to cellulite formation, which means having your levels checked. Insulin, adrenal hormones, prolactin and hormones produced by the thyroid all act to produce cellulite. Estrogen may be a major factor involved as well, though studies are still being done to determine its full impact. Abnormal levels in any of these hormones could be a cause of your cellulite.

200.   One of the best things you can do about cellulite is to watch what you eat. You need to eat a diet that has less processed foods and fats and more fiber, fruit and vegetables. Foods with chemicals preservatives and such are not able to be fully flushed from your body.

201.   Use moisturizer daily. While moisturizer won't all of a sudden cure you from cellulite, what it will do is plump up your skin and make it look healthier. It'll hydrate you, and that leads to

less of that cellulite being seen when you are out in public. Try moisturizing twice a day, once right after a shower.

202.   Want long lasting results that make your cellulite disappear? Getting a massage can tighten up the bumps in your thighs. Whether it's a professional massage or a friend or family member, a massage is a great way to help out.

203.   Make positive lifestyle changes to reduce your cellulite or prevent it. Even though there are cosmetic cellulite products out there, they aren't proven to be completely effective. Exercising and eating healthy keeps hormones at bay. Avoid stress and anything that will impact your hormone cycle.

204.   If using squats to combat cellulite, be sure you are doing them at least three times per week. You should be doing at least fifteen squats per workout to ensure the best results. If you can do more, go for it! The tighter your legs are, the leaner they will look.

205.   Reducing stress can help reduce cellulite. Stress causes you hormones to be affected. Then your body starts producing stress hormones like cortisol which can affect your appetite and the

way that your body metabolizes things. So try to keep stress at a manageable level and have ways to deal with it when it does appear.

206.   Lecithin is an important nutrient for skin health. Apples, lettuce, and soy beans are rich in lecithin, so try to work them into your diet. A salad with these ingredients can make for a good lunch if you want to be healthy.

207.   Reduce your salt intake. Salt causes you to retain fluids and many of those fluids retain toxins. Reducing your salt intake is one of the best ways to keep you body's ability to continually flush itself of toxins. Drink tea instead as it a natural diuretic and has many other health benefits.

208.   Do not buy any creams that promise to help you get rid of cellulite because these things never work. The only things these products may offer is a temporary reprieve. You should keep your money in your pocket because any who offers a miracle cure is out to scam you.

209.   Do not believe the myth that cardio is the best way to get rid of cellulite. While it does work to some degree, you have to combine it with other exercises. This will not totally remove

any cellulite in the body, but it will definitely improve the way it looks.

210.   To hide cellulite and battle it at the same time, try some Slendesse leggings. These leggings are made to give you the appearance of firmness that you so desire. And they do much more! They are actually made with both shea butter and caffeine right in the fibers themselves. This helps battle the cellulite for real while you wear them.

211.   A better diet can help you in your battle with cellulite. You should be consuming enough vegetables and fruits daily. Doing this creates an alkaline ash which can reduce the appearance of cellulite, among other things. Juicing is a great way to get the amount of fruits and vegetables that you need as well.

212.   Green tea is a great tool in your battle against cellulite. It contains many great ingredients that can help boost the body's fat-pocket breaking abilities. That, of course, means less cellulite. You can get green tea capsules if you prefer because they are more potent.

213.   Both men and women can have cellulite, but women are more likely to be affected by it. The reason for this may be partly hormonal, or it may

be the result of the type of fat and connective tissue females typically have. The condition is not well understood, and more research is required.

214.   Physical exertion is a great way to get rid of cellulite. For starters, when you workout or do any kind of physical activity, you are sweating out harmful toxins that can be causing cellulite. Also, certain exercises can tighten up the areas where you have cellulite, reducing the appearance of cellulite.

215.   To reduce the appearance of cellulite, make sure you exercise on a regular basis. Make sure you work up a good sweat when you exercise. Sweating helps expel toxins from the body through the skin. Exercise also improves your body's appearance by toning and tightening, so you look better even if you have cellulite.

216.   Some methods that have been used to remove cellulite include heat therapy, pneumatic massages, ultrasound and electrical stimulation. Unfortunately, none of these methods have been proven to work. Probably the most effective way to get rid of cellulite is to eat nutritious, low fat foods that are high in fiber. This causes weight loss and reduction of fat.

217.   You can fight off cellulite by using creams and products that contain caffeine. You can not get the same results by drinking a lot of coffee or other beverages that have caffeine. Using caffeinated beauty products can keep skin tighter for hours. The caffeine in them works by temporarily eliminating the connective tissue's water. This makes any dents in the skin less noticeable.

218.   Poor blood circulation could be a contributing factor to your cellulite. Avoid sitting for extended periods of time. If you must sit for work, try to get up at least every half hour for five minutes or so. That will get the blood flowing and will reduce the effects that cellulite has on your buttocks and upper thighs.

219.   Try to cut down the stress you're experiencing, or learn to deal with it in a positive way. When you are stressed out, your cortisol levels increase. Cortisol is known as the "stress hormone", and when cortisol goes up, you increase your ability to store fat. Cortisol is also linked to thin skin, so if you want to improve your skin, you need to learn to deal with the stressors you have.

220.   Use caffeine filled body scrubs on the areas of your body in which cellulite is a problem. These scrubs can help to break up any fatty deposits in the area causing you the problems. Look for an exfoliator that has caffeine, avocado oil and can be used generously in the area.

221.   When looking at your cellulite problem, it is important to know if you have a genetic predisposition. Gender plays the major part; however, factors such as race, metabolic rate and circulatory issues are involved as well. Being genetically susceptible to cellulite will have an impact on your approach to prevention.

222.   Cellulite may be less noticeable if you get a tan. Cellulite doesn't look quite so bad when it's darker. It is important that you begin with skin exfoliation to help smooth the skin's surface by using a good body scrub, then apply the tanning lotion.

223.   Take a look at what you're using for contraception. Is it hormonal contraception? Contraception that influences your hormone levels is a big cause of considerable weight gain and cellulite for a lot of women. If this is a problem for you, you may want to consider discussing alternatives with your doctor.

224.   A soothing massage can be a fantastic way to minimize your cellulite! The kneading action is great for circulation, and can improve the streng

225.   Apply moisturizer often. Keeping skin moisturized is great for lots of reasons. It really does help fight cellulite. When applying lotion, massage your problematic areas daily. The massaging motion can reduce cellulite by breaking up the deposits of fat under the skin.

226.   Try bursts of intensive exercise to lower those cellulite fat deposits. A good exercise to do this with is jumping rope. Keep the exercise short and intense helps target those areas you are having trouble with, while not disrupting your day. Try to find a few minutes every few hours and get a few repetitions in.

227.   A natural way to get rid of cellulite is by switching your salt. Believe it or not, table salt could be causing you to have cellulite; its acidity depletes you of minerals you need in your body. It makes your body more "toxic." Switch over to Himalayan crystal salt or Celtic sea salt.

228.   Cellulite may be caused by poor diet choices that are high in fat, salt, carbohydrates and

minimal fiber. People who smoke, do not exercise enough and sit or stand for extended periods of time are also more likely to develop cellulite. Genetics may also make some people predisposed to the condition.

229.   Get rid of the anxiety in your life to beat cellulite. When a stressful situation occurs, the hormone Cortisol is let loose in your body. It can thin the skin and increase the fat storage in your body. Meditation and yoga are great techniques for relieving the stress you are dealing with.

230.   You can fight off cellulite by using creams and products that contain caffeine. You can not get the same results by drinking a lot of coffee or other beverages that have caffeine. Using caffeinated beauty products can keep skin tighter for hours. The caffeine in them works by temporarily eliminating the connective tissue's water. This makes any dents in the skin less noticeable.

231.   Try to stay active and avoid erratic dieting. Many people like to hit the diet hard, meaning they are very aggressive with their program. These sudden and major changes in your body can impact hormone production, as well as confusing your system. Avoid diets that suggest

major changes to diet and activity immediately, if cellulite is a concern.

232.   Use a moisturizer. However, try not to fall victim to claims of miracle results. There is no one product that is going to get rid of all your cellulite, all on its own. Still, a moisturizer is important, and you should try and select something that was designed to target cellulite.

233.   You can try using bronzer to fight off your cellulite. A faux tan in the area that are prone to tan make your skin look better and draw attention away from the dimples. The darker colors can make these dimples appear smaller. Just make sure to exfoliate first with a gentle body scrub on those areas, then you can use a tanning lotion or spray.

234.   To reduce the toxins that worsen the appearance of cellulite, give your trouble areas a massage everyday. You can use massage tools, brushes, or even specially shaped soaps to give yourself the massage. The massage will stimulate your circulatory and lymphatic systems which will help move toxins out of the areas you target.

235.   Want to get rid of that pesky cellulite? Rub some coffee grounds into the area. Give it a

good, deep massage and allow the coffee to exfoliate the top layers of skin. Add a little olive oil for lubrication and to ensure the coffee doesn't just fall off all over your floor.

236.   Drink enough clean water. This will help you to flush toxins and extra sodium in your system. When you have extra sodium in your body and retain water, that can eventually cause cellulite. Drinking enough water will help you to avoid those dimples. If you don't like water, you can flavor it as well.

237.   To make your exercise regime help you battle against cellulite, don't forget the squats. This will help to get blood to the area, puffing it up and making the lumps less visible. On top of that, toned legs always look more taut. Lastly, you'll be burning the fat which causes the cellulite in the first place.

238.   If you want a temporary quick-fix to reducing you cellulite, apply a caffeine-based cream to your skin. Caffeine temporarily gets rid of water in the connective tissues, reducing the dimple appearance in the skin. Before applying the cream, make sure you exfoliate with a body scrub or loofah to maximize the effects of the cream.

239.   Because there is no cure for cellulite and it is hereditary, the only thing you can do is attempt to cover it up. Using self tanner, especially if you are pale, can reduce the appearance of dimpled skin on your legs and buttocks. Self tanner is also a relatively inexpensive product!

240.   Massaging your cellulite with exfoliating scrubs or a massager with knobs can break up the fat and distribute it more evenly. You can also try using self tanner or serums made to make your skin look smoother. There is no magical formula for busting cellulite, but these can certainly help.

241.   If all other solutions fail, you may want to consider liposuction to battle cellulite. This is an serious medical treatment, so it should not be the first thing you go to. And it's not foolproof, as some cellulite can actually look worse after liposuction. Weigh your options carefully and talk with your doctor.

242.   If you have cellulite that you have been trying to get rid of, you should try getting more exercise. While this will not make the cellulite go away, it will redistribute some of the fatty deposits and remove some of the excess fluids.

This will make the problem areas look a lot smoother.

243.   Try bursts of intensive exercise to lower those cellulite fat deposits. A good exercise to do this with is jumping rope. Keep the exercise short and intense helps target those areas you are having trouble with, while not disrupting your day. Try to find a few minutes every few hours and get a few repetitions in.

244.   Cut down on the salt that you eat in your diet. Salt may taste good, but it actually makes you retain fluids. This can be very problematic and increase cellulite pockets. If you lower the amount of salt you eat, you could see a surprising amount of improvement quite quickly.

245.   Make sure that you're drinking plenty of water. There are many reasons to drink water. When you're not drinking enough water, sodium can build up. This can cause you to retain water, producing excess cellulite. Drinking plenty of water can remedy this and keep your skin hydrated, cutting down on cellulite.

246.   Cellulite does not discriminate. Regardless of whether you are overweight or thin, you have the potential to get cellulite. Still, the heavier you are,

the worse the cellulite will look on you. As a result, it is important to establish a regular exercise regimen in order to minimize the appearance of the cellulite.

247.   If you have cellulite in your thigh region, you should get into cycling. Go for a long bike ride a few times a week. When your legs pump the pedals, your thigh muscles work and burn off the fat in that region. You will notice that your thighs will begin to look leaner and firmer.

248.   Realize that cellulite doesn't mean you have to lose weight, or that you are not healthy. A lot of women have cellulite, including famous people, and there isn't much to do to rid your body of it. Don't feel bad about a normal part of life.

249.   You can try using bronzer to fight off your cellulite. A faux tan in the area that are prone to tan make your skin look better and draw attention away from the dimples. The darker colors can make these dimples appear smaller. Just make sure to exfoliate first with a gentle body scrub on those areas, then you can use a tanning lotion or spray.

250.   Use moisturizer daily. While moisturizer won't all of a sudden cure you from cellulite, what it will do is plump up your skin and make it look healthier. It'll hydrate you, and that leads to less of that cellulite being seen when you are out in public. Try moisturizing twice a day, once right after a shower.

251.   Do you want to find ways to keep cellulite off of your body? Massage your skin to make the bumps disappear. The results are not permanent, but will remain for several days.

252.   You can help banish cellulite by not smoking. Smoking introduces toxins into your body. Those toxins interfere with your ability to easily flush your body and reduce the blood flow to areas of your body. Smoking also adds wrinkles to your face so it is something that you should never do anyway.

253.   If using squats to combat cellulite, be sure you are doing them at least three times per week. You should be doing at least fifteen squats per workout to ensure the best results. If you can do more, go for it! The tighter your legs are, the leaner they will look.

254.   If you're self conscious about your cellulite while working out, try wearing shorts that are made to make your legs and buttocks appear slimmer. Some shorts even contain caffeine and enzymes that are included to reduce the appearance of dimpling once you are doing working out and take off the shorts.

255.   When it comes to combating any fat, cardio is your best friend. When you exercise, be it riding a bike, going for a swim or hitting the gym, you're burning fat. The more fat you burn, the tighter your body will become. To get rid of cellulite, boost your heart rate!

256.   Try giving yourself a massage if you have trouble areas. That massage a few times a day can really help break down the cellulite that's present. Massaging helps bring more blood flow to these areas. This will aiding in thickening the skin and making cellulite less noticeable.

257.   Change the types of fruits you eat. You may be thinking you're doing the right thing eating bananas, mangos and grapes, but those are actually relatively fattening fruits. If you change over to fruits in the berry family - like blueberries and strawberries - you'll consume a lot less calories. That means less cellulite too.

258.   To get the most out of your diet, eat lots of high fiber foods like vegetables and whole grains. The faster you flush toxins from your body, the better you will feel and look. Go for items which are low in sugar, such as celery, citrus and even the tasty plum.

259.   Try eating more essential fatty acids to keep cellulite at bay. They can help strengthen your skin's connective tissues that surround fat cells, which helps reduce cellulite. Diet that containing essential fatty acids helps the fat cells from slackening, which can reduce the dimpling. Some products that contain these fatty acids are flaxseed oil, olive oil, walnut oil, blackcurrent seed oil, and fish oil.

260.   Boost the amount of water you drink to win the battle with your cellulite. Staying hydrated may not cure cellulite, but it can stop it from occurring or reoccurring. Maintaining proper skin hydration is very essential. This also helps get rid of toxins from your system. Drink at least 6 glasses of water a day.

261.   Dehydration is not your friend, and it certainly does you no favors when it comes to cellulite. Get up each morning and reach for a

glass of water. Carry a water bottle with you throughout the day so that you remember to continue drinking. And, stay away from things like coffee, which can have a dehydrating effect.

262.   Pick up a cellulite mitt and work on your troubled areas from right inside your home. Cellulite mitts have raised ridges and knobs that help promote circulation and blood flow when you scrub your body with them. This then helps your body break down those pockets of ugly cellulite.

263.   If your diet is good, you can get rid of cellulite and also stop it from happening. In particular, add foods that have lecithin. Some foods with lecithin include peanuts, eggs, apples and lettuce. In addition, avoid very fatty foods.

264.   Minimize the appearance of cellulite by limiting the amount of skin thinning cream you use. Using skin thinning creams, like steroid, on areas of cellulite will make the cellulite more obvious. This is due to your skin being thinner and making the dimples under your skin more noticeable. Also, any imperfections in the skin will be more visible.

265.   Add more fatty acids to your diet in order to reduce cellulite. They help to make connective tissue around your fat cells stronger. Also, they help to slow down the production of fat cells, thus reducing cellulite. Good sources of fatty acids include blackcurrent seed oil, olive oil, fish oil, and flackseed oil.

266.   Cellulite is often the result of accumulated toxins within the body. Therefore, to really start eliminating the condition and the bumpy appearance everyone dreads, embark on a clean diet of unprocessed foods and fresh water. It will not be long at all until the cellulite starts to become a distant memory.

267.   Do you want to get real, enduring results in your fight against cellulite? A massage may be one of the best ways to help those lumpy thighs appear tighter. You can either enjoy a day at the spa, or coax your hubby to give you a massage, but the results will be evident for several days.

268.   Try moisturizing and massaging your skin to fight off cellulite. Skin needs an extra hand from time to time. Help it by moisturizing it. Then, break down its fatty cells via kneading in the areas that are prone to cellulite. Combining these two methods tens to be effective. To boost

results, apply moisturizer in a circular motion to boost circulation and cut down on fatty deposits.

269. Take up swimming to burn cellulite! Studies have shown that swimming for an hour two or three times a week can not only burn fat, but melt away cellulite as well. This is because the water micro-massages your skin as you swim. Start slowly and gradually build up to a good hour long anti-cellulite workout.

270. Avoid smoking. Smoking inhibits your body's capacity to resolve toxins. This can cause issues with cellulite because the skin loses its elasticity. Find a way to eliminate smoking from your life in order to fight cellulite, as well as to improve your overall health.

271. When it comes to combating any fat, cardio is your best friend. When you exercise, be it riding a bike, going for a swim or hitting the gym, you're burning fat. The more fat you burn, the tighter your body will become. To get rid of cellulite, boost your heart rate!

272. The gym offers many ways for you to exercise, but focus on the cardio machines if your goal is to beat cellulite. For example, running on a treadmill, biking on a recumbent

bicycle or even hitting the elliptical can get your heart pumping. The harder you work, the more fat you will shed.

273.   Alternate your showers between hot and cold. When you're showering, try switching to cool water for a few minutes and then back to hot. Go back and forth a few times as you shower. This can really do wonders for the circulation in your skin, which can help get rid of cellulite.

274.   Follow a comprehensive detox plan. A thorough cleansing and detox will work wonders for your body. There are many ways you can go about this; you simply need to find one that is suitable. Your body can work more effectively to fight cellulite when the toxins are flushed from your system.

275.   Break up the fat deposits under your skin and distribute them more evenly with massage. If you don't have the money for scrubs or soaps containing caffeine, you can use a regular knobbed massager. This not only feels good, but it will make your legs appear smoother and tighter, too!

276.   You have to ensure that you consume plenty of fatty acids. It's not the case that you should keep away from all fats; these acids are a must. They actually help you minimize the amount of cellulite on your body. It is important to look for healthy ways to consume those essential fatty acids.

277.   If you have cellulite that you have been trying to get rid of, you should try getting more exercise. While this will not make the cellulite go away, it will redistribute some of the fatty deposits and remove some of the excess fluids. This will make the problem areas look a lot smoother.

278.   Try using a body brush on your skin. Brushing your skin with a body brush is a great way to reduce cellulite. It removes dead skin cells and stimulates blood flow. Brush your problem areas in an upward direction to break up fatty deposits and cut down on some of that unsightly cellulite.

279.   Drink lots of water. This is the easiest and really most effective thing that you can do to battle cellulite. If you get eight glasses per day into your diet, that water will help get toxins out

of your body. Plus it'll pump up your circulation too. All of which will lead to less cellulite.

280.   As you probably already know, cellulite is fat. If you are carrying excess weight on your body, this may be the reason why you have cellulite. One way to remedy this problem is by engaging in some form of physical exercise several times each week. Some excellent choices are swimming, running, jogging, walking and yoga.

281.   Cellulite may be caused by poor diet choices that are high in fat, salt, carbohydrates and minimal fiber. People who smoke, do not exercise enough and sit or stand for extended periods of time are also more likely to develop cellulite. Genetics may also make some people predisposed to the condition.

282.   If you actively smoke, give up the habit as quickly as you can. Smoking only makes cellulite worse. Smoking introduces toxins, which make your skin less flexible and tougher. That will make cellulite worse. In time, wrinkling and dryness will occur as well. If you can't quit on your own you may want to speak with a doctor for more assistance.

283.   Increasing your activity level can be a big help in the fight against cellulite. Cardio classes, strength training and even brisk walking all help to burn the fat that goes into making that ugly cellulite on your thighs. Increase exercises that tone your thighs to keep your skin elastic and smooth.

284.   Cutting down on your stress can also help you reduce your cellulite. When you have stress, the "stress hormone" cortisol is released into your body. Cortisol not only makes your body store more fat, but also makes your skin thinner. Meditation and yoga are both great things to do if you're dealing with stress.

285.   If you have got problems with cellulite, consider cutting down on your daily sugar intake. Sugar is a primary cause of cellulite, because it creates a build up of fat in your body. This leaves you with those unsightly dimples that are so difficult to get rid of! Cut down on sugar and loose cellulite.

286.   If you have cellulite in your thigh region, you should get into cycling. Go for a long bike ride a few times a week. When your legs pump the pedals, your thigh muscles work and burn off the

fat in that region. You will notice that your thighs will begin to look leaner and firmer.

287.   Because cellulite normally appears on the thighs, legs, and buttocks, try toning these areas. Lunges and squats are easy exercises you can do anywhere to strengthen these areas. Building up the muscle can help to alleviate the appearance of the fat deposits that can appear underneath the skin to create cellulite.

288.   Try to stay active and avoid erratic dieting. Many people like to hit the diet hard, meaning they are very aggressive with their program. These sudden and major changes in your body can impact hormone production, as well as confusing your system. Avoid diets that suggest major changes to diet and activity immediately, if cellulite is a concern.

289.   Consider adding Murad's Firming and Toning serum to your beauty regime. It doesn't just have caffeine, but also includes a few more ingredients which make it a one-two punch for skin care. It has cayenne, for example, which helps to stimulate the skin's blood flow, improving its look and quality.

290.	Try adding more oily fish to your diet if you are having difficulty getting rid of cellulite on your body. Consuming fish that is rich in unsaturated Omega-3 oil, such as trout or tuna, is a proven way to minimize cellulite. Make sure you prepare it in a healthy way too, like baked or on a salad.

291.	Poor blood circulation could be a contributing factor to your cellulite. Avoid sitting for extended periods of time. If you must sit for work, try to get up at least every half hour for five minutes or so. That will get the blood flowing and will reduce the effects that cellulite has on your buttocks and upper thighs.

292.	Use moisturizer daily. While moisturizer won't all of a sudden cure you from cellulite, what it will do is plump up your skin and make it look healthier. It'll hydrate you, and that leads to less of that cellulite being seen when you are out in public. Try moisturizing twice a day, once right after a shower.

293.	Diet to lose weight. This is an obvious one, but still needs to be stated. Cellulite is essentially cured by getting into better shape and a healthier weight. It may mean a complete change in how you approach your food, but it can really be worth it to look your best.

294.   Cardo exercises are one way that you can bring your cellulite under control. If you regularly exercise and try targeting areas with cellulite, you can beat it. Biking and running are great exercises to improve your thighs, hips, and buttocks.

295.   Do not buy any creams that promise to help you get rid of cellulite because these things never work. The only things these products may offer is a temporary reprieve. You should keep your money in your pocket because any who offers a miracle cure is out to scam you.

296.   To reduce the amount of cellulite you see on your body, try applying a firming gel at least once a day. This type of gel helps firm and tone those areas, so there's less of those fatty deposits to see. A good time to use it is right after you leave the shower in the morning.

297.   Try wearing "Tonewalker" sandals to fight that cellulite. These sandals actually are designed to help make your muscles work a lot harder while walking. This in turn firms your muscles and combats that unsightly cellulite! It's an

amazing benefit. Just think - every step that you take will actually help you combat those areas.

298.   Stay away from refined salt. It will dehydrate you and take valuable minerals from your body. Sea salt is a much better option, as it is good for your body and has a pleasing flavor as well. Most people do not even notice a difference in the two, so the switch should not affect you very much.

299.   As you probably already know, cellulite is fat. If you are carrying excess weight on your body, this may be the reason why you have cellulite. One way to remedy this problem is by engaging in some form of physical exercise several times each week. Some excellent choices are swimming, running, jogging, walking and yoga.

300.   To keep cellulite at bay, try maintaining a regular exercise regimen that includes lunges. These particular moves really help firm up the thighs. These exercise build up lean muscle in the thighs and buttocks, which cellulite is generally present. Maintain proper form when doing these exercises to keep away the cellulite by not letting your knees go too far over your toes. Also, keep the heel on the front foot pressed into the floor while squeezing your glutes.

301.   Since cellulite can be caused by wearing tight fitting garments around the waist and lower body, it is best to wear clothing that does not bind and reduce circulation. Some people wear compression garments to minimize the lumpy appearance of the condition. This may minimize the bumpy appearance, but does not correct the problem.

302.   Water is very important to beating cellulite. The more you drink, the more supple your skin will be. Hydration will keep you skin taut and also flushes toxins. As a result, your skin will look great!

303.   Try to stay active and avoid erratic dieting. Many people like to hit the diet hard, meaning they are very aggressive with their program. These sudden and major changes in your body can impact hormone production, as well as confusing your system. Avoid diets that suggest major changes to diet and activity immediately, if cellulite is a concern.

304.   One of the best things you can do about cellulite is to watch what you eat. You need to eat a diet that has less processed foods and fats and more fiber, fruit and vegetables. Foods with

chemicals preservatives and such are not able to be fully flushed from your body.

305.   Water is essential in keeping your body looking lean, but do not drink too much. Excess water can make you feel bloated, and it can result in swelling under the cellulite. Drink no more than one and one-half liters for the optimal hydration of your body without over doing it.

306.   If you have dark skin and bronzer doesn't show up well on your legs, use body oil on the front of your thighs to draw the eye away from the cellulite on the back. Everyone is like a little bird, their eye drawn to bright and shiny things, so use it to your advantage.

307.   In the battle against cellulite, many people have found real success with the multiple formulations of topical treatment available on market. However, the key to getting lasting results lies within commitment and routine. When applied religiously on a daily basis, it is possible to see a change sooner than you may have thought possible.

308.   Try to cut down the stress you're experiencing, or learn to deal with it in a positive way. When you are stressed out, your cortisol

levels increase. Cortisol is known as the "stress hormone", and when cortisol goes up, you increase your ability to store fat. Cortisol is also linked to thin skin, so if you want to improve your skin, you need to learn to deal with the stressors you have.

309.   If all other solutions fail, you may want to consider liposuction to battle cellulite. This is an serious medical treatment, so it should not be the first thing you go to. And it's not foolproof, as some cellulite can actually look worse after liposuction. Weigh your options carefully and talk with your doctor.

310.   There are some creams which help with cellulite, but they are often best used in conjunction with the other tips listed here. In fact, even the cheapest Nivea firming cream offers great benefits when paired with massage, eating the right foods and exercise. Check reviews online to see what the latest, greatest creams happen to be.